The Solution For Managing Blood Sugar THE SOLUTION FOR

MANAGING BLOOD

SUGAR

Diet And Nutrition

Nikki M. Vara

1

The Solution For Managing Blood Sugar Table of content

<u>Introduction</u>

Chapter1 1
body control blood sugar? 1
What is blood glucose? Moreover, how does the 1
Understanding Blood Sugar..1
Foods to Include and Avoid...4

CHANGES IN DIET TO MANAGE BLOOD SUGAR.....................4
Chapter 2...4
Hydration...7
Sample Meal Plans: Choices for Breakfast 9
Chapter 3...9
Exercise, relaxation, and stress reduction................................14
MANAGEMENT 14
LIFESTYLE CHANGES FOR BLOOD SUGAR 14
Chapter 4...14
Stress Management...15
Sleep 16
Vitality of Monitoring 18
Monitoring and tracking blood sugar 18
Chapter 5...18
Techniques for checking blood sugar 19
Blood sugar tracking and recording...19
Conclusion 20
Chapter 6...20

3

The Solution For Managing Blood Sugar Introduction

Eating three meals a day at regular intervals is the foundation of a diabetes diet. This improves how well you use the insulin your body makes or receives from a medicine. A diabetes diet's primary objective is to maintain blood sugar levels in a healthy range while also enhancing general health and well-being.

You can create a diet based on your health objectives, preferences, and lifestyle with the assistance of a trained dietitian. Also, he or she can advise you on how to change your eating patterns, such as by picking portions that are appropriate for your size and level of activity.

Use these nutrient-dense meals to make your calories count. Choose wholesome carbohydrates, foods high in fiber, seafood, and "good" fats. Foods rich in monounsaturated and polyunsaturated fats can lower your cholesterol levels, making them good fats. They consist of:

Avocados, nuts, and oils such as canola, olive, and peanut Bringing everything together to come up with a plan To assist you to maintain a normal blood glucose level, you can develop a diabetes diet using a number of different strategies. A diabetes diet generally entails choosing healthful foods and keeping an eye on portion sizes to help 4

The Solution For Managing Blood Sugar control blood sugar levels and lower the risk of problems related to diabetes.

Chapter1

Understanding Blood Sugar

What is blood glucose? Moreover, how does the body control blood sugar?

A type of sugar that circulates in the circulation and gives energy to all of the body's cells is known as blood sugar, commonly referred to as blood glucose. The majority of the body's cells and organs get their energy from it. Our bodies convert carbs, such as those found in bread, pasta, and fruit, into glucose when we eat them. The body's cells utilize this glucose as fuel after it is absorbed into the bloodstream and delivered there. A hormone called insulin, which is created by the pancreas, signals cells to take up glucose from the bloodstream, assisting in the control of blood sugar levels. Insulin aids in maintaining healthy blood sugar levels, preventing them from getting too high or too low.

5

The Solution For Managing Blood Sugar Blood sugar levels can rise too high if the body doesn't create enough insulin or if cells start to resist it.

Hyperglycemia is the name of the disorder, which can cause diabetes, heart disease, and nerve damage, among other health issues. It's crucial for overall health and well-being to monitor blood sugar levels and keep them within a healthy range.

Blood sugar levels are controlled by a sophisticated system within the body that involves the interplay of numerous hormones and organs.

Carbohydrates are converted into glucose when we eat them, which is then released into the bloodstream. This causes the production of insulin from the pancreas, a hormone that facilitates

1

the movement of glucose from the bloodstream into our body's cells for use as energy.

If blood sugar levels go too low, the pancreas releases glucagon, which tells the liver to release glucose from storage into the bloodstream to bring them back up.

Other hormones, such as cortisol and adrenaline, can impact blood sugar levels in addition to insulin and glucagon. For instance, the stress hormone cortisol, which is secreted, can raise blood sugar levels by prompting the liver to release glucose from storage into the blood.

Physical activity, dietary preferences, and medicine all have an impact on the body's capacity to control blood 6

The Solution For Managing Blood Sugar sugar levels. People can boost their body's capacity to control blood sugar levels by choosing healthy lifestyle habits including frequent physical activity and a balanced diet and maintaining overall health. How the Body Reacts to Blood Sugar

Blood glucose, often known as blood sugar, is crucial in giving our body's cells energy.

However, having blood sugar levels that are either too high or too low might be harmful to our health.

The eyes, kidneys, neurons, blood arteries, and other organs and tissues can become damaged when blood sugar levels are too high, as is the situation with uncontrolled diabetes. Over time, issues like heart disease, stroke, renal disease, and nerve damage are more likely to occur due to high blood sugar levels. Having low blood sugar, sometimes referred to as hypoglycemia, can be risky. Confusion, drowsiness, trembling, and in severe cases, loss of consciousness, are all signs of hypoglycemia. Hypoglycemia can occasionally be brought on by overusing diabetes medications, missing meals, or indulging in vigorous exercise without consuming enough calories.

Chronic changes in blood sugar levels can have long-term negative impacts on our health in addition to these immediate ones. Prolonged exposure to high blood sugar levels, for instance, has been linked to oxidative stress, inflammation, and cellular damage, all of which have been found to raise the chance of developing chronic 7

The Solution For Managing Blood Sugar conditions including type 2 diabetes, cardiovascular disease, and cancer. Hence, it's crucial for overall health and lowering the risk of complications related to diabetes to maintain optimal blood sugar levels through food, exercise, and medication control.

Type 1 diabetes and Type 2 diabetes are the two types of the disease.

The cells in the pancreas that make insulin, a hormone that aids in controlling blood sugar levels, are attacked and destroyed in Type 1 diabetes by the immune system. In order to control their blood sugar levels, persons with type 1 diabetes need insulin injections or an insulin pump.

When Type 2 diabetes develops, the body becomes less responsive to the effects of insulin, and the pancreas may not be able to generate enough of the hormone to maintain healthy blood sugar levels. The management of type 2

diabetes frequently involves dietary and activity modifications, as well as the use of blood sugar-lowering medicines. If left unchecked, both types of diabetes can have harmful repercussions on the body. The eyes, kidneys, nerves, and blood arteries are just a few of the organs and tissues that elevated blood sugar levels can harm over time. Complications include heart disease, stroke, kidney disease, and nerve damage may result from this. Complications include heart disease, stroke, kidney disease, and nerve damage may result from this. Diabetes can also lead to other issues like foot issues, skin diseases, 8

The Solution For Managing Blood Sugar dental issues, hearing loss, and sleep apnea. Also, those who have diabetes are more likely to contract infections, particularly those that affect the skin, gums, and feet. To prevent or manage any potential complications, it is crucial for people with diabetes to closely monitor their blood sugar levels and work with their healthcare team to create a personalized management plan that includes a healthy diet, regular physical activity, medications, and regular check-ups.

Chapter 2

CHANGES IN DIET TO MANAGE

BLOOD SUGAR

Foods to Include and Avoid

Avoiding meals that can spike blood sugar levels quickly is crucial for controlling blood sugar or diabetes.

Examples of foods to limit or stay away from are as follows:

Sugary beverages: Due to their high sugar content, drinks including soda, sweetened tea, and fruit juice can quickly raise blood sugar levels.

Foods that have been processed and packaged: A lot of processed and packaged foods have additional sugars, 9

The Solution For Managing Blood Sugar refined carbs, and bad fats that can increase blood sugar levels.

These foods—white bread, pasta, and rice—are made from refined carbohydrates, which can quickly raise blood sugar levels. Use whole-grain alternatives instead.

Desserts and sweets: Candy, cakes, cookies, and other sweets should be consumed in moderation or avoided due to their high sugar content.

Foods that are fried or heavy in fat can lead to inflammation and insulin resistance, which can make it more difficult to control blood sugar levels.

processed and red meats,

enormous amounts of food Egg yolks, liver, and other organ meats are sources of cholesterol, as are high-fat dairy products, high-fat animal proteins, and these foods.

Strive to consume no more than 200 mg of cholesterol each day.

Focus on eating a balanced diet instead, one that consists of full, unprocessed foods like fruits, vegetables, whole grains, lean meats, and healthy fats. These meals offer crucial nutrients for overall health and can assist in balancing blood sugar levels. Working with a healthcare practitioner to create a custom dietary plan that suits every person's needs and tastes is also crucial. foods to mention It's crucial to concentrate on consuming nutrient-dense foods that are high in fiber, protein, and healthy fats while controlling blood sugar levels or managing diabetes 10

The Solution For Managing Blood Sugar through dietary modifications. The following foods can be incorporated into a diabetic or blood sugar diet: veggies without grains: Leafy greens, broccoli, cauliflower, bell peppers, and carrots are a few of these.

They have a lot of fiber, are rich in nutrients, and have few calories.

Brown rice, quinoa, whole wheat bread, and oats are examples of whole grains. They include a lot of fiber, which can aid in reducing the rate at which sugar is absorbed into the body. Simple carbohydrates like sugars and complex carbs like starches are broken down during digestion to produce blood glucose.

Chicken, turkey, fish, tofu, and legumes like beans and lentils are examples of lean protein. Protein can maintain fullness and help control blood sugar levels.

Olive oil, almonds, seeds, avocados, and other healthy fats are examples. They can lessen inflammation and aid insulin sensitivity. Monounsaturated and polyunsaturated fatty acid-rich foods can aid in lowering your cholesterol levels. But, limit your intake because all fats are high in calories.

Dairy products with low-fat content include milk, yogurt, and cheese. Although they are good providers of protein and calcium, take note that flavored variants often contain additional carbohydrates. Fruits: They can still be a part of a balanced blood sugar or diabetic diet but should be consumed in moderation due to their natural sugar 11

The Solution For Managing Blood Sugar content. Choose foods with a low glycemic index, like berries, apples, and citrus fruits.

Spices and herbs can flavor food without adding additional calories or sugar. Examples include ginger, turmeric, and cinnamon, which have been demonstrated to potentially reduce blood sugar levels.

Also, it's crucial to minimize or stay away from meals like processed foods, sugary beverages, and refined carbs that might raise blood sugar levels. A specialized meal plan can be made by working with a registered dietitian or other healthcare professionals to address specific requirements and objectives. Controlling portions and timing meals

To prevent overeating and maintain steady blood sugar levels throughout the day, portion control is a crucial component of blood sugar management. Here are some suggestions for controlling portions while controlling blood sugar:

Use more compact plates: Making servings appear larger and encouraging lesser portion amounts can both be accomplished by using smaller plates.

Count and weigh the food: To guarantee proper serving sizes, use measuring cups, food scales, or portion control plates.

Recognize how to gauge serving sizes: You can eventually develop the skill of estimating portion sizes by utilizing your hand or other visual cues. For instance, a 12

The Solution For Managing Blood Sugar serving of cheese is roughly the size of a small matchbox, whereas a serving of cooked veggies is roughly the size of your fist. Examine food labels to learn about serving sizes and nutritional information about foods. When choosing foods, pay attention to the portion size and total carbs.

Non-starchy vegetables should make up half of your plate: Non-starchy vegetables with low-calorie counts and high fiber content, like leafy greens, broccoli, and cauliflower, can help you feel full and control blood sugar levels.

Limit foods high in carbohydrates: Carbohydrate-rich foods can quickly cause blood sugar levels to rise. To help slow down the absorption of sugar into the bloodstream, it's crucial to choose sensible serving amounts and combine them with protein and healthy fats. Meal timing is an important aspect of managing blood sugar levels.

Here are some tips for meal timing when managing blood sugar:

Don't skip meals: Skipping meals can cause blood sugar levels to drop too low, which can lead to feelings of fatigue, dizziness, and irritability. It can also cause overeating later in the day.

Eat at regular intervals: Eating at regular intervals can help keep blood sugar levels stable. Aim to eat three meals a day and add healthy snacks if needed.

Eat breakfast: Eating breakfast can help kickstart your metabolism and prevent overeating later in the day.

Choose a breakfast that is high in fiber and protein, such 13

The Solution For Managing Blood Sugar as oatmeal with nuts and berries or eggs with whole-grain toast.

Give your body time to digest and metabolize the food between meals by spacing them out by at least 2-3 hours.

Take medications and meal timing into account: See your doctor about the optimal time to take your blood sugar-regulating drugs with meals if you take them. It may be necessary to take some drugs with food and others on an empty stomach.

Be cautious when munching at night: Avoid eating too close before going to bed because this can raise blood sugar levels and interfere with sleep. If you feel like you need a snack, go for something small and low in carbohydrates, such as a piece of cheese or a handful of almonds. Remember, everyone's needs are different, so it's important to work with a registered dietitian or healthcare provider to develop a personalized meal plan that meets your individual needs and goals.

Hydration

Staying hydrated is important for managing blood sugar levels. Here are some hydration tips when managing blood sugar:

Drink plenty of water: Water is the best choice for staying hydrated. Aim for at least 8-10 cups of water per day.

14

The Solution For Managing Blood Sugar Avoid sugary drinks: Sugary drinks, such as soda, juice, and sweetened tea, can cause blood sugar levels to spike.

Choose water, unsweetened tea, or flavored water instead.

Alcohol should not be consumed on an empty stomach since it can cause blood sugar levels to drop too low. If you decide to consume alcohol, do it moderately and with meals.

Sports drinks and energy drinks are two examples of beverages that may contain hidden sources of sugar.

Carefully read the labels before selecting low- or sugar-containing choices.

While exercising or perspiring a lot, you might need to replace any electrolytes that were lost through sweat. To assist replenish electrolytes, think about consuming coconut water or a sports beverage with reduced sugar.

Remember that everyone has different needs, so it's crucial to collaborate with a registered dietitian or other healthcare professionals to create a customized food and hydration plan that suits your needs and goals.

15

The Solution For Managing Blood Sugar Chapter 3

Sample Meal Plans: Choices for Breakfast

This is an example of a healthy breakfast to control blood sugar levels:

Nuts and Berries in Oatmeal:

Rolling oats in a cup, half

1 cup of unsweetened almond milk a half-cup of berries (such as strawberries, blueberries, and raspberries)

1/fourth cup of chopped nuts (such as almonds, walnuts, or pecans)

Instructions:

To add more protein and flavor, add unsweetened almond milk instead of water when cooking the oats according to the directions on the package. Add chopped nuts and mixed berries to the cooked oats as a garnish.

Serving hot, please.

The Solution For Managing Blood Sugar The substantial fiber, protein, and healthy fat content of this breakfast option can help maintain stable blood sugar levels throughout the morning. The nuts lend a pleasant crunch, added protein, and good fats, while the berries offer natural sweetness and antioxidants. To help you stay full and content until your next meal, be sure to serve this breakfast with a source of lean protein, such as a boiled egg or Greek yogurt.

Option 2: Egg and avocado toast Whole-grain bread, one slice

1/4 mashed avocado

1 cooked or poached egg

Olive oil, 1 teaspoon

To taste, add salt and pepper.

Instructions:

When desired, toast the bread.

Olive oil should be heated in a small pan over medium heat. Cook the egg to your taste after cracking it into the pan (e.g. poached or boiled).

Add salt and pepper and spread the mashed avocado across the toast.

The fried egg is placed on top of the avocado toast.

These choices are rich in fiber, protein, and healthy fats, which can help control blood sugar levels and keep you feeling content and full.

Smoothie, third choice

The Solution For Managing Blood Sugar Smoothie: A smoothie made with frozen berries, unsweetened almond milk, and a scoop of protein powder can make for a filling and blood sugar-friendly breakfast option.

Meal Schedule

These are some illustrations of lunch menus: 1st Lunch Plan:

Salad with grilled chicken: Mixed greens, cherry tomatoes, cucumbers, sliced avocado, and a dressing of olive oil and balsamic vinegar.

Sliced strawberries, blueberries, and raspberries for dessert are examples of fresh fruit.

Quinoa and veggie bowl for Meal Plan 2: roasted sweet potatoes, cooked quinoa, sautéed spinach, and chickpeas with a tahini dressing drizzle.

Greek yogurt: Plain Greek yogurt sprinkled with cinnamon and topped with finely chopped almonds for extra crunch and protein.

Meal Plan 3: Turkey Wrap: A whole-grain wrap stuffed with diced turkey breast, mixed greens, diced tomatoes, and avocado, with a honey mustard dressing drizzled on top.

Carrots and hummus: A crunchy, high-fiber snack of carrot sticks and hummus.

18

The Solution For Managing Blood Sugar Lentil soup from the fourth meal plan is created from scratch with a variety of vegetables, including celery, onions, and carrots. Served with whole-wheat toast.

Apple slices: For a sweet and filling dessert, combine sliced apples with almond butter or peanut butter.

Meal Plan 5: Tuna salad sandwich: Greek yogurt, diced celery, red onion, canned tuna, and whole-grain bread are combined to make the tuna salad.

Roasted vegetables: Carrots, broccoli, and cauliflower roasted with garlic and olive oil.

Keep in mind to modify these meal plans to suit your nutritional requirements and tastes.

dinner choice

These are some examples of supper menus: Option 1: Grilled salmon. Season salmon with black pepper, garlic, and lemon juice before grilling it until it is fully cooked.

Quinoa salad: Prepare the quinoa as directed on the package, then combine it with the mixed greens, cucumber, cherry tomatoes, and a mild vinaigrette dressing.

Option 2: Baked chicken. To prepare, season chicken breasts with a blend of dried herbs and spices before baking them in the oven.

19

The Solution For Managing Blood Sugar Vegetables roasted in the oven until tender: Mix your favorite vegetables, such as broccoli, cauliflower, and carrots, with olive oil.

Option 3: Beef stir-fry: In a pan, sauté beef strips with garlic, ginger, and soy sauce until the meat is fully cooked.

Bell peppers, onions, and snap peas are a few of your favorite stir-fry vegetables that you can include.

Cook brown rice as directed on the package instructions and serve alongside the stir fry Option 4: Vegetarian chili: In a pot, cook bell peppers, onions, and garlic until they are soft. Stir in the kidney beans, black beans, cumin, chili powder, and canned tomatoes, and cook for 20 to 30 minutes.

Making a batch of cornbread to go with the chili is simple.

Option 5: Vegetable and shrimp skewers: Vegetables like zucchini, bell peppers, and cherry tomatoes can also be skewered with shrimp and grilled until thoroughly cooked.

Quinoa pilaf: Prepare quinoa as directed on the package, then mix in sautéed onions, garlic, and your preferred herbs and spices.

Note that these are only representative evening menus and that you should adjust your meal plan to suit your particular dietary requirements and tastes.

20

The Solution For Managing Blood Sugar Snack choices

When controlling blood sugar, it's crucial to select snacks that are low in refined carbohydrates and added sugars, as these might lead to blood sugar rises. Although these can help control blood sugar levels, choose snacks that are heavy in fiber, protein, and healthy fats instead.

Here are a few examples of snack menus and snacks to help you control your blood sugar: Example snack strategies

Plan 1:

A single tiny apple and one tablespoon of almond butter one boiled egg

ten young carrots and hummus

Plan 2: 1/4 cup of fresh berries, 1/2 cup of unsweetened Greek yogurt, and 1 tablespoon of chopped almonds.

Sliced cucumbers and 2 tablespoons of hummus on a single small whole-grain pita

1 small pear along with 1 ounce of cheese Plan 3:

with 1/4 cup of cherry tomatoes and 1 tiny avocado Edamame in a cup

a single little banana and a single tablespoon of peanut butter

Snack Selections

21

The Solution For Managing Blood Sugar Try munching on carrot sticks, cucumber slices, or bell pepper strips while dipping them in a dish of hummus.

Almonds, walnuts, pumpkin seeds, and sunflower seeds are all rich sources of protein and good fats. To avoid overeating, keep in mind that nuts and seeds might contain a lot of calories.

Hard-boiled eggs: Hard-boiled eggs are a good source of protein and can be a satisfying snack on their own or paired with veggies.

Fresh fruit: Apples, bananas, and berries are all great options for a quick and easy snack.

Cheese: A small serving of cheese can provide protein and healthy fats. Try pairing it with whole-grain crackers or sliced veggies.

Remember, it's important to talk to your healthcare provider or a registered dietitian about a personalized plan for managing your blood sugar levels.

22

The Solution For Managing Blood Sugar Chapter 4

LIFESTYLE CHANGES FOR BLOOD

SUGAR MANAGEMENT

Exercise, relaxation, and stress reduction Frequent exercise can help lower systolic blood sugar (the top number) by an average of 4 to 9 mm Hg, making it a beneficial lifestyle adjustment for controlling blood sugar.

Moreover, exercise can help to strengthen your heart and enhance your cardiovascular health in general. Adults should perform at least 150 minutes of moderate-intensity aerobic activity or 75 minutes of vigorous-intensity aerobic activity per week, according to the American Heart Association. This can involve exercising vigorously, such as running, cycling, swimming, or walking.

Here are some pointers on how to incorporate exercise into your daily routine to control your blood sugar:

• Begin slowly and build up the length and intensity of your workouts over time.

• Choose a workout you can stick with and like.

• Vary your workouts to keep them exciting and difficult.

• To keep motivated, think about hiring a personal trainer or enrolling in a group exercise program.

23

The Solution For Managing Blood Sugar

• Include strength training workouts in your regimen to increase muscle mass and your level of fitness.

• Schedule exercise into your calendar to make it a regular part of your day.

• Check your blood pressure frequently to track how an activity is affecting your health.

Never begin an exercise regimen without first talking to your doctor, especially if you have a medical issue like high blood sugar or any underlying ailment.

Stress Management

Stress can have a significant impact on blood sugar levels in individuals with diabetes. Therefore, managing stress is an essential part of managing blood sugar levels. Here are some lifestyle changes that can help with stress management:

·

Exercise regularly: Regular exercise can help reduce stress and improve blood sugar control. Aim for at least 30 minutes of moderate-intensity exercise most days of the week.

·

Practice relaxation techniques: Techniques such as deep breathing, meditation, and yoga can help reduce stress and promote relaxation.

·

Get enough sleep: Lack of sleep can lead to increased stress levels and blood sugar fluctuations. Aim for 7-8 hours of sleep per night.

24

The Solution For Managing Blood Sugar

·

Limit caffeine and alcohol: Caffeine and alcohol can both increase stress levels, so it's best to limit or avoid them altogether.

• Look for support: Speaking with loved ones or a mental health expert can help you better control your stress and enhance your general well-being.

• Control your workload: Setting priorities, assigning chores to others, and establishing attainable goals can all help you feel less stressed and avoid burnout.

• Make time for fun activities: Taking part in hobbies or other enjoyable pursuits can help you feel better and reduce stress.

But keep in mind that finding what works best for you is a continuous process. Don't lose hope, be patient, and don't be afraid to ask for assistance if you need it.

Sleep

In particular, for those with diabetes, getting adequate sleep is crucial for maintaining blood sugar levels. These are some lifestyle modifications you may do to enhance your sleep and assist in blood sugar control:

• Create a consistent sleeping schedule: Try to go to bed and get up at the same times every day, even on the weekends.

25

The Solution For Managing Blood Sugar

• Establish a calming sleep ritual, which can include taking a warm bath, reading a book, or engaging in relaxation exercises like deep breathing.

• Don't use electronic gadgets just before bed: The blue light they emit can interfere with your sleep, so it's best to put them away at least an hour before you go to bed.

• Avoid caffeine and alcohol: These two substances should be avoided, especially in the evening, as they can both interfere with your ability to fall asleep.

Maintain a cold, quiet, and dark bedroom: Make sure your bedroom is comfortable for sleeping by maintaining these conditions.

• Engage in regular exercise: Exercise can help you sleep better and lower your blood sugar levels.

• Control stress: Stress can affect your sleep and cause blood sugar levels to rise, so it's crucial to discover methods of controlling stress, such as through meditation, yoga, or other relaxation techniques.

You can enhance your sleep and assist control your blood sugar levels by changing your way of living. But if you still have issues sleeping or controlling your blood sugar, it's crucial to talk to your health provider 26

The Solution For Managing Blood Sugar Chapter 5

Monitoring and tracking blood sugar Vitality of Monitoring

To effectively control diabetes, blood sugar levels must be monitored. These are some justifications for why it's crucial:

Keeping problems at bay Over time, having high blood sugar levels can cause major health issues like heart disease, kidney damage, nerve damage, and eyesight loss.

The early detection of elevated blood sugar levels made possible by routine monitoring can help avoid these problems.

Changing the course of treatment: By keeping track of blood sugar levels, diabetic patients and their medical professionals can modify their regimens of medication and lifestyle modifications including food and exercise.

Monitoring blood sugar levels regularly can help discover patterns of high or low readings, which can assist people with diabetes in making the required modifications to their treatment plan.

Monitoring blood sugar levels can assist diabetics in taking an active role in their health and in developing better self-management techniques.

The Solution For Managing Blood Sugar Individual empowerment: Knowing their blood sugar levels can assist people with diabetes make wise decisions about their lifestyle and health.

It's crucial to collaborate with a healthcare professional to decide how frequently blood sugar levels should be checked and what goal values are suitable for a person's particular circumstances.

Techniques for checking blood sugar There are numerous ways to check blood sugar levels, including:

The most popular way to check blood sugar levels at home is through self-monitoring of blood glucose (SMBG). In SMBG, the quantity of glucose in a drop of blood taken from a fingerstick is measured using a glucose meter.

Depending on the person's needs and the healthcare provider's suggestions, the frequency of testing varies.

• Continuous glucose monitoring (CGM): This technique includes wearing a tiny sensor beneath the skin to continuously monitor glucose levels all day and all night.

The sensor wirelessly transmits information to a receiver or smartphone, which shows the glucose readings and gives alerts when levels are too high or low.

• Hemoglobin A1C (HbA1C) testing: This blood test gauges your average blood sugar levels over the previous two to three months. It is advised for persons with diabetes 28

The Solution For Managing Blood Sugar to get it at least twice a year to assess long-term glucose control.

• Urine glucose testing: This technique involves checking for the presence of glucose in the urine. However, it is not advised as the main way of monitoring because it is less accurate than SMBG or HbA1C tests.

The ideal way to monitor your blood sugar levels should be discussed with your healthcare professional because the frequency and type of tests may differ based on the demands and medical background of the individual.

Blood sugar tracking and recording An essential component of managing diabetes is monitoring and recording blood sugar levels. Here are a few techniques for doing that: 1. A blood glucose logbook is a physical or digital record of blood glucose readings that are taken throughout the day. Information about meals, exercise, medicine, and other notes pertinent to managing diabetes can also be recorded in the diary. A logbook can be made by downloading and printing readings from a built-in memory that some glucose meters have.

2. Apps for tracking blood sugar levels, medication, meals, physical activity, and other diabetes-related data are widely available for smartphones and other mobile devices. Several of these apps can sync with glucose meters and offer information and tailored advice.

29

The Solution For Managing Blood Sugar 3. Electronic health records (EHRs): Accessible by healthcare professionals, EHRs are electronic versions of a patient's medical records. During office visits or remotely through patient portals, blood glucose measurements, and other diabetes-related data can be input into the EHR.

4. Continuous glucose monitoring (CGM): As was already mentioned, CGM devices continuously measure blood sugar levels and can be used to identify patterns and trends over time. You and your healthcare practitioner can use the data to download and evaluate it to make educated decisions about managing your diabetes.

Whatever the approach, it's critical to constantly record and monitor blood sugar levels to see trends, choose the best course of therapy, and interact with medical professionals.

Chapter 6

Conclusion

For several reasons, getting medical advice on blood sugar is crucial. For one thing, only a qualified medical 30

The Solution For Managing Blood Sugar professional can accurately diagnose diabetes and other conditions linked to blood sugar. It's crucial to get medical counsel if you think your blood sugar levels may be high or low to identify the underlying problem and the best course of action. To avoid problems, blood sugar-related diseases need to be managed and treated continuously. A healthcare professional can create a personalized treatment plan for you that may include medication, lifestyle modifications, and blood sugar level monitoring.

However, prolonged high blood sugar levels might result in consequences like nerve, kidney, and eye damage.

The early detection and management of these issues through routine medical checkups can assist to stop them from getting worse. A healthcare professional can offer guidance on controlling blood sugar levels as well as advice on stress reduction, physical activity, and healthy food. Also, they can offer assistance and resources for coping with the emotional effects of having a blood sugar-related disease.

In general, consulting with a doctor about blood sugar is essential for precise diagnosis, efficient treatment and control, monitoring for problems, and receiving support and education.

Changing Your Nutrition to Empower Yourself Making dietary changes can help you control your blood sugar levels. Here are some pointers: Choose complex carbohydrates: Meals abundant in fiber, like whole grains, fruits, and vegetables, can aid in 31

The Solution For Managing Blood Sugar reducing the pace at which sugar is absorbed into the bloodstream, preventing blood sugar increases.

Limit your portion sizes: Consuming too much of any food might raise your blood sugar levels. To guarantee proper servings, use measuring cups or a food scale.

Minimize additional sugars since processed foods and sugary beverages can raise blood sugar levels. Opt for low-sugar liquids like water or unsweetened tea instead.

Minimize your intake of sweets and desserts, and choose items sweetened naturally with things like fruit.

Emphasize protein and healthy fats: Good fats, including those in nuts, seeds, and avocados, can help reduce the rate at which sugar is absorbed into the bloodstream.

Protein can also keep the blood sugar level stable. Eat frequently since skipping meals or waiting too long between them might cause blood sugar levels to spike or fall uncontrollably. Include regular meals and snacks in your daily routine.

A registered nutritionist should be consulted: Personalized advice and assistance on controlling blood sugar levels through dietary adjustments can be obtained from a licensed dietitian.

Making dietary adjustments to control blood sugar levels can be empowering, but it's crucial to collaborate with a healthcare professional to make sure that these adjustments are suitable and safe for each person's needs and medical background.

32

The Solution For Managing Blood Sugar 33